Reflexology for Beginners!
How to Take Charge of Your Health, Happiness and Well-Being

By

Indiana Standfield

Table of Contents

Copyright

What Is Reflexology?

Reflexology is a gentle therapeutic technique of restoring the body's balance and relieving pain. This unique method is a non-invasive procedure geared towards relaxation, stress relief, and pain alleviation. It works through the controlled stimulation of various pressure points on certain areas of the body – feet, hands, and ears. It is in these areas that the imbalances are addressed in order to maintain homeostasis, or the body's natural balance and equilibrium.

The principle behind reflexology lies on the concept that the body's organs and glands can be mapped through nerves scattered onto the different reflex areas. Predefined pressure points, located in the reflex areas, are stimulated by means of specific reflexology techniques. These areas are sensitive and need utmost care when handled. Too much pressure exerted to the reflex areas may cause discomfort for some patients. As such, it is highly recommended for patients to consult a practitioner to ensure safety on one's health.

A practitioner of reflexology is an individual who is trained to carry out reflexology techniques to patients. Practitioners of reflexology include reflexologists, chiropractors, massage therapists, physical therapists, and others. Practitioners make use of body charts as a guide in locating the areas where pressure must be applied. Some practitioners use rubber balls, wooden sticks, or bands in applying pressure. However, the hands and fingers are commonly used in finding and working through each tensed and congested pressure points.

The practice of reflexology is increasing in popularity because of its effectiveness in relieving pain and stress, improving blood circulation, bringing relaxation, and other benefits. Studies have also shown that reflexology may aid in reducing psychologically-related conditions such as severe anxiety and depression. Reflexology is also used as a complementary treatment to other health therapies to speed up the healing process. Additionally, reflexology promotes holistic healthcare for the prevention of some illnesses.

Where Does Reflexology Come from?

The origin of reflexology can be traced way back to ancient Egyptian times. The first recorded accounts of reflexology can be found in pictographs on Ankhamor's Egyptian tomb, dated 2330 BC. In 2450 BC, a Sixth Dynasty Egyptian tomb has walls showing two men massaging their hands and feet.

Reflexology is also said to have originated from pre-dynastic China and ancient India. Symbols depicting the practice of reflexology can be seen on the feet of the statues of Buddha. The Yellow Emperor's Classic of Internal Medicine, a Chinese medicine manual written in 1000 BC, has a single chapter dedicated to the importance of examining one's foot and its relation with the body's functions. From then, the practice of reflexology was passed on through oral tradition – leading to its development in European and Native American cultures.

In recent times, it was Dr. William H. Fitzgerald who introduced reflexology in the United States. Thus, Dr. Fitzgerald was referred to as the Father of Reflexology. In 1917, Dr. Fitzgerald wrote about the ten vertical zones found in the body. These vertical zones are extended from the head up to the tips of the fingers and toes. According to him, applying sufficient pressure into these zones could bring about pain relief in the injured parts of the body – a concept also known as zone analgesia or zone therapy.

Another prominent figure in the development of reflexology is Dr. Shelby Riley. He did further studies on Dr. Fitzgerald's work by introducing the horizontal zones in the body. He developed a detailed map of the reflex points located at the feet and hands. Dr. Riley was the first to determine the various pressure points on the ears.

Eunice Ingham, a colleague to Dr. Riley,

discovered the pressure points in the feet and the corresponding organs they affect. It was through her research, in 1930, where it was found out that the feet possess the most sensitive and responsive pressure points. Ms. Ingham was also responsible for the development of the modern foot maps and reflexology charts still used today. The reflexology maps for the ears were developed by Dr. Paul Nogier in 1957. Ms. Ingham's nephew and niece, Dwight Byers and Eusebia Messenger, founded the National Institute of Reflexology in 1968. In the early 1970s, this institute was renamed the International Institute of Reflexology.

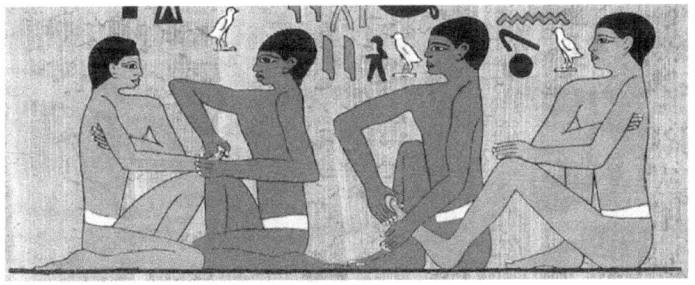

Source:
http://www.reflexologyroomlondon.co.uk/history-of-reflexology

Principles Surrounding Reflexology

The main principle surrounding the practice of reflexology is that when stress is released, the body will eventually achieve its natural stability and balance. When this happens, the body will be able to regenerate and heal itself. There are, however, a number of theories explaining how reflexology works. All of these theories are integral in the development of the modern practice of reflexology.

The theory stating the correlation of reflexology with the central nervous system is the most prominent one. This theory was postulated through the research conducted by Sir Henry Head and Sir Charles Sherrington in the 1890s. Based on their research, the skin and the internal organs are shown to have a neurological relationship between them.

It is due to this relationship that the process of any reflexology session stems from. The pressure applied into the reflexology areas – feet, hands, and ears – serves as a stimulus for the peripheral nerves found in these areas. Such stimulus is transferred into the central nervous system which would enable the necessary adjustments in the body.

Another theory of reflexology is called the Gate Control Theory, or more commonly known as the Neuromatrix Theory of Pain. The gist of this theory is that reflexology can cause pain relief through stress reduction and mood improvement. This theory states that pain is a subjective experience of the brain. Pain is created as the brain's response to a sensory input or emotional and cognitive stimuli.

In reflexology, it is believed that the human body consists of both a physical and emotional aspect. The practice of reflexology is geared towards overall healing – physical body, mind, and spirit. This means that the body can only obtain relaxation if both the mind and spirit are in a calm state.

Lastly, there is a theory explaining that the constant flow of vital energy into the body is the key to the body's wellness. If a person is experiencing stress, the vital energy is congested and the energy flow is blocked. This energy congestion is perceived as the cause of various illnesses and abnormalities. As such, the application of pressure into the reflexology areas promote continuous energy flow.

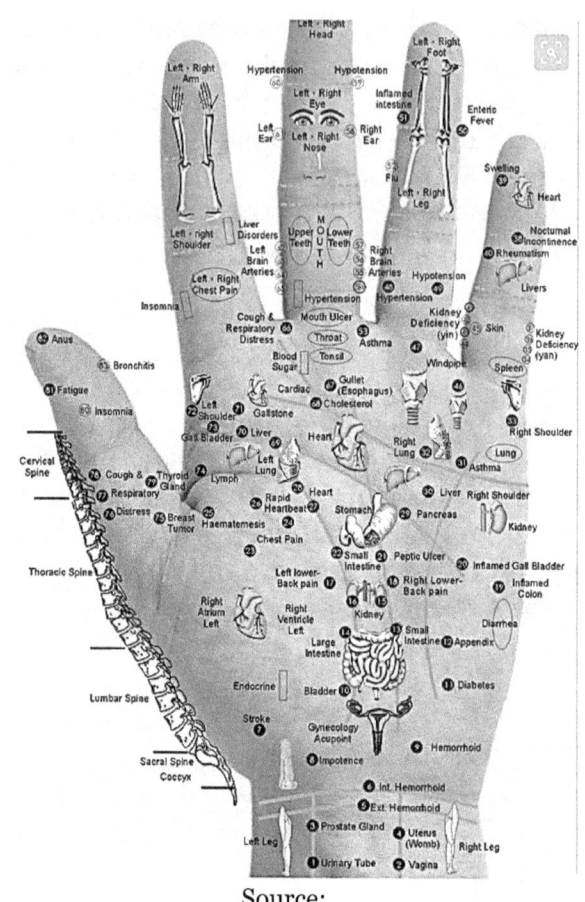

Source:
https://au.pinterest.com/pin/455708056015456773/

Where Are the Reflexology Points and Areas?

In general, the reflexology points and areas in the body are on the feet, hands, and ears. It is in these areas where nerves – directly connected to specific organs, glands, and body systems – are located. These reflexology areas are targeted by practitioners in order to correct any discomfort or imbalances within the body.

The pressure points are widely spread throughout the reflexology areas. For the feet and hands, the pressure points are accessed through the bottom, top, and the sides. The ears have pressure points both on the outer and inner parts. Using the finger to reach into the ear's inner part can access these points.

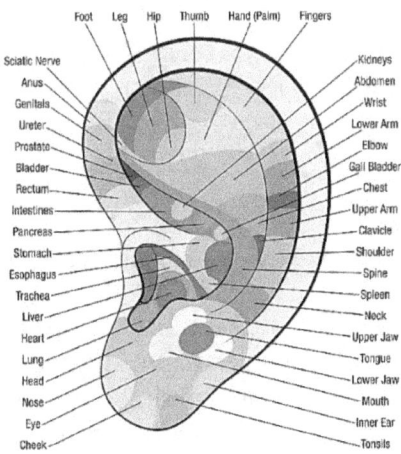

Ear Reflexology Chart

In reflexology, practitioners make use of reflexology maps in order to distinguish which pressure points correspond to which internal organs. These maps also serve as a guide to know which areas are in need of attention.

The foot reflexology map is the most commonly used map for the practice of reflexology. In this map, it is noticeable that each foot corresponds to one vertical half of the body. The left foot is connected to the left side of the body – including all organs, glands, and others. Consequently, the right foot is connected to the right side of the body.

FOOT MASSAGE CHART

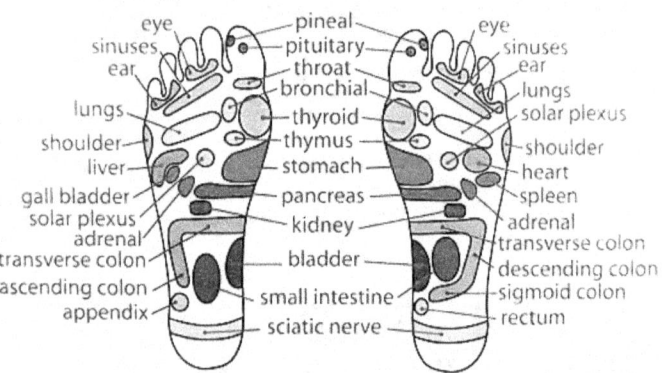

Source: http://www.trinity-nhc.com/Reflexology.html

When undergoing reflexology, both the hands, feet, and ears can be focused on simultaneously. The practitioner should work on de-stressing certain parts of the body through touching and massaging.

Hand Reflexology Chart

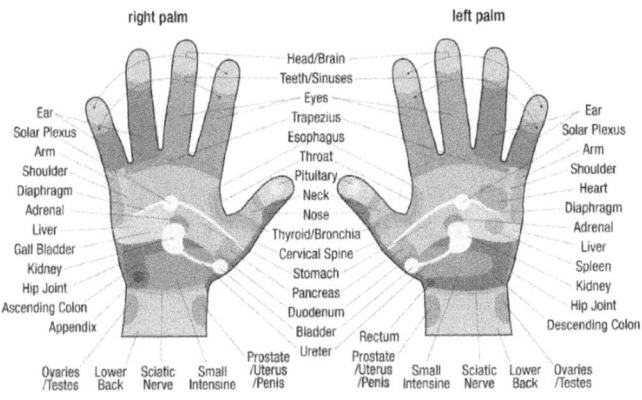

Source: https://bio-sources.com/reflexology-insoles/

Head Reflexology Chart

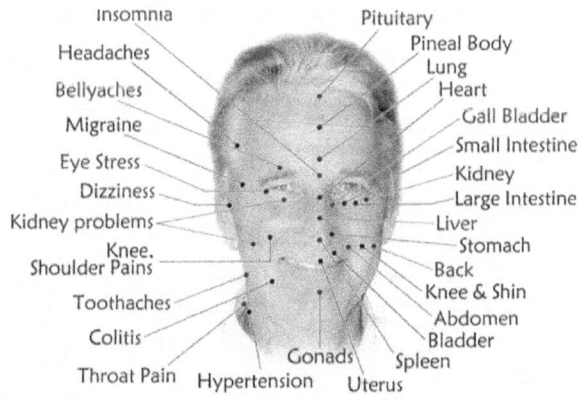

Source: https://s-media-cache-ako.pinimg.com/564x/cd/3d/43/cd3d43960f3e363891cc17d7f87fc733.jp

How Does Reflexology Relate to Other Therapies?

Reflexology is loosely related to most therapies and relaxation techniques. More often than not, reflexology is practiced as a complement to other therapies in order to fully promote healing. Furthermore, reflexology brings about various health benefits as with other therapies.

The principle used in reflexology is similar to that of acupuncture and acupressure. Both types of therapies make use of the stimulation of specific points in the body in order to enhance the body's condition. Additionally, these "points", both used in reflexology and acupuncture, are quite similar in such a way that they affect other parts of the body when stimulated.

However, the points for acupuncture or acupressure do not always coincide with the points for reflexology. The reflex points for reflexology are only found in the feet, hands, and ears. These points are in arrangement depending on which organs they are connected to. On the other hand, the points used for acupuncture are arranged along thin energy lines in the body, called meridians.

It is a common mistake to confuse reflexology with massage. People should know that these terms are not interchangeable. The only thing that makes them alike is the use of touch to carry out the therapy. However, their approach differs greatly from each other. Massage is the handling of the body's tissues and muscles, in a systematic way. It uses various massaging techniques – kneading, stroking, and rubbing – in order to provide relaxation directly into the affected muscles and limbs. On the other hand, reflexology uses the exertion of subtle pressure on specific points and areas of the body. These points are handled using delicate hand and finger techniques – thumb and finger walking – in order to affect several parts throughout the body.

Massage works in releasing pain and tension when pressure is exerted on specific muscle groups. Reflexology stimulates the nerves, located in the pressure points, in order to release tension. Simply put, massage focuses on spot correction while reflexology has holistic benefits.

Your first Reflexology visit

Here is a thorough guide on how a typical reflexology appointment goes. This is helpful for first timers to know what they should expect on their first reflexology visit. Common concerns about reflexology are also addressed in this section.

What Happens Before the Session?

A reflexology session does not start with the touching of the reflex points right away. It has to start with an in-depth evaluation of the patient's overall health and condition. The practitioner should first conduct a health and lifestyle consultation on the patient before proceeding with the therapy.

Reflexology is a form of therapy which manipulates sensitive and highly responsive nerves in the body. As such, it is important for the practitioner to evaluate the patient's overall health. The patient will be asked a series of questions regarding his medical history, especially for the first treatment, to check if the patient is suitable for a reflexology session. The patient should disclose any recent medications, surgeries, and other medical conditions. If the patient is deemed unfit for this type of therapy, he will not be allowed to undergo the therapy. There are certain health conditions which are not allowed for those who will undergo a reflexology session – which will be discussed in the next chapters.

The reflexology practitioner will give the patient an overview of the reflexology session. The feet and hands are to be examined by the reflexologist. The patient should be reminded that reflexology does not treat or diagnose any illnesses. It also should not serve as a substitute therapy and treatment for any medical condition.

By this time, the patient is given an opportunity to ask any questions or concerns, if he has any. It is important for the patient to gain enough information about the reflexology session he is about to experience. It is absolutely normal for the patient to feel nervous towards the session, especially for first timers. However, communication with the reflexologist will certainly put any patient at ease.

Lastly, the patient is asked to sign a waiver or form of consent before proceeding with the reflexology session. All personal information should be kept confidential.

What Happens During the Session?
Unlike having a massage, the patient is not asked to take off their clothes during reflexology. Gloves, socks, shoes, and other apparel covering the hands and feet are the only articles of clothing required to be removed. Otherwise, the patient should wear loose and comfortable clothes to induce relaxation.

The practitioner could play some relaxing music to create a healing environment. Scented candles and oils may be used to add tranquility with the treatment's ambiance. Throughout the reflexology session, the practitioner should always stay present whilst exhibiting a calm and relaxed state.

The reflexology session may focus on the feet, hands, ears, or on all three – depending on the specific health concerns that the patient has. The practitioner should inform the patient about the focus of the reflexology session and the course of treatments recommended.

The reflexologist will have to focus carefully on the specific area corresponding to the health problem which the patient needs improvement upon. However, the reflexologist should work on the entire area with gentle pressure. The reflexologist should work on all reflex points in order to address all organs, glands, and nerves. Doing so will allow any congestions on the nerve pathways to be released and promote relaxation. As the session starts, the patient may be asked to lie on a couch or sit down. The patient should maintain this relaxed position throughout the session. The feet, hands, and ears are then washed and soaked in lukewarm water. The reflexologist will assess the area of focus for any skin conditions – open wounds, sores, rashes, and skin allergies – and current pains. Having these abnormal conditions are prohibited during reflexology.

The treatment starts with gentle pressures applied on the reflex points. The reflexologist may use a cream or powder to help the fingers work their way through the reflexology area. The pressure applied on the patient should be firm, but gentle, and not vigorous – so as not to inflict pain.

The session starts at either the patient's toes or fingers, working through the heel, and ending at the sides and top of the feet or hands. If any pain or tightness is found, the reflexologist will work continuously on the area until harmony and balance is brought about. In reflexology, it is only through restoring the body's balance that the pain can be released. The practitioner may return to these areas throughout the session to make sure that the pain is gone.

Usually, a reflexology session lasts 30 to 60 minutes. It is allowed for the patient to take a nap or chat during the whole session, whichever he prefers. For first timers, it is important to know that it is quite normal to feel a bit of discomfort during their first treatment. However, the whole experience should be relaxing. If the patient feels that the discomfort is intolerable, he can request the practitioner to stop at any time.

Generally, patients feel a sense of relaxation and rest. Some experience a warm, tingling sensation throughout their body. Energy movement is also felt in the specific body area being worked on. Patients may also feel light-headed, relaxed muscles, and drowsy.

What Happens at the End of each Session?

At the end of the session, the reflexologist may stroke the patient's hands and feet to wrap it up. Doing so will help the patient feel nurtured and cared for. The reflexologist may recommend the patient to drink water and rest a bit. The patient should take his time to compose himself after the session. Alcohol and excessive food intake are prohibited every after a complete session.

The practitioner should take notes regarding the session. This will help the practitioner in determining the improvements needed for any future appointments. Additionally, these notes will help the practitioner to fully customize succeeding sessions to meet the patient's needs.

Any changes in the body will be noticeable after a few reflexology sessions. Various effects may arise after the treatment. Most patients experience total relaxation and sense of well-being. Others, however, experience feelings of lethargy and nausea. These bodily reactions are actually parts of the patient's healing process. They are indications that the body is returning to homeostasis, or the body's state of balance and harmony.

These reactions include:
- Improved energy and stamina
- Improved sleep
- Pain and tension relief
- Fatigue and drowsiness to enable the body to rest
- Skin breakouts, rashes, and pimples caused by the release of toxins and impurities
- Diarrhea and frequent bowel movements due to cleaning and detox
- Increased discharge of mucus
- Emotional and psychological relief which includes being tearful and emotionally-sensitive

To date, the practice of reflexology does not have known negative side effects. Any inconveniences experienced after the treatment are caused by the elimination of toxins from the body. Increased water intake reduces the severity of these inconveniences and maximizes the benefits received.

How Many Reflexology Sessions Are Needed?

The number of sessions needed depends on the patient's current health condition. To get the maximum benefits of reflexology, it is recommended to have regular appointments – one session a week for about 4 to 6 weeks. Short sessions, which are done frequently, are recommended to speed up the body's process of healing. Nevertheless, reflexology sessions can be done as frequent as the patient desires.

If a patient has a specific health condition or illness, more frequent reflexology sessions is recommended – once a week for 6 to 8 weeks would suffice. After the weekly appointments, the frequency of treatment may be reduced to one session per month.

Limitations of Reflexology
Reflexology is used in keeping the body in harmony and balance. It is perceived that the body will eventually repair itself from inconsistencies once the stress from the body is released. Reflexology cannot be used to diagnose any illnesses based on observed tension or congestion in the reflexology areas.

If a reflexologist encounters abnormalities during the session, he should suggest for the patient to seek assistance from a medical professional. The reflexologist is, in no way, authorized to give diagnosis or any medical advice regarding the patient's health condition. Additionally, reflexologists are not allowed to prescribe any type of medication to patients. Reflexology is used to complement any therapy which a patient is currently undergoing – not to replace it.

When to avoid Reflexology

Reflexology is an absolutely safe form of therapy which could be administered to anyone, in a general manner. In fact, even babies and toddlers could benefit from this form of therapy. However, there are a few instances wherein a patient is not allowed to have a reflexology session. It is important to consider these precautions first before getting an appointment.

Reflexology is not suitable for patients with unhealed and open wounds, rashes, and other severe skin conditions. Undergoing a reflexology session could only worsen the current skin condition of the patient.

The foot is the most effective, yet most sensitive, reflexology area. As such, patients with foot fractures and foot gout are not allowed to go through reflexology. Patients suffering from osteoarthritis affecting the foot area and vascular disease of the legs and feet are considered unsuitable for foot reflexology. In case a patient has health concerns regarding the feet area, he should get a consultation with a medical professional first. Reflexology on the hands or the ears is the best alternative for this situation.

Patients suffering from embolism or thrombosis are discouraged from undergoing reflexology treatment. Reflexology will regulate the circulation of blood into the body. Doing so could contribute to aggravating the situation by pushing the blood clot into the heart or brain.

Pregnant women are highly vulnerable to illnesses, although the reflexologist may customize the therapy based on the needs of a pregnant woman. The reflex points linked to the uterus and ovaries are either addressed gently or totally avoided in order to avoid any complications. However, there is still a chance that overstimulation of a certain reflex point could cause contractions. As such, pregnant women should be careful when undergoing reflexology regardless of the alteration of the treatment.

Patients with chronic or severe diseases need permission from a medical personnel before going to a reflexologist.

Although reflexology works as a complement to other forms of therapies, a patient still needs to take precautions so as not to worsen the current illness.

Lastly, people who have other forms of therapies need to allot enough time before going to a reflexology session. An interval of at least 48 hours is needed in between therapies. This time allowance will avoid too much fatigue on the body caused by the various therapy sessions.

What Are the Benefits of Reflexology?

Different forms of therapy promise a number of health benefits. In general, reflexology focuses on improving the body's internal organs in order for them to function properly. Although these benefits are still insufficiently proven, there have been some cases reporting the wonders that reflexology can give. Here are some of the important benefits of reflexology.

Relaxation and Stress Reduction

One of the most prominent benefits of reflexology include relaxation and stress reduction. Reflexology aids in the continuous flow of vital energy in the body. Through this, any stress in the body is released, leading to a secured balance in the body.

The results vary for each patient. In most cases, however, reflexology is known to provide soothing relaxation and comfort.

Pain Reduction

In line with relaxation, reflexology is also proven to reduce the severity of bodily pain and tension. In fact, it is one of the primary reasons so many people opt for reflexology. Thumb and finger walking in a certain reflex area can ease out any blockage, which causes pain, in the pathway of vital energy. A session of reflexology therapy promotes balance in life and body – enforcing pain reduction.

Reflexology is also effective in combating severe headaches and migraine. This form of therapy is especially effective for stress-induced headaches. Coupled with proper medication, people experience great improvements in their condition and lessened episodes of migraines when they start having reflexology. Additionally, the symptoms for migraine and severe headache are reduced.

Improved Nerve Function

Nerve endings decrease in performance as people age. The nerve endings become less responsive and less sensitive to stimulus. When this happens, the nervous system will have a difficulty in interpreting any input coming from the nerve endings. This could bring a huge impact on the performance of the different organs in the body. Through reflexology, these nerve endings are highly stimulated and repaired. The pressure applied on the reflex points will clean out the neural pathways within the body. This enhances optimum functioning to the internal organs. Reflexology can also speed up cognitive learning, memory, and mental reactions.

Regulate Blood Circulation

A single session of reflexology can bring significant improvement in blood circulation. With proper circulation, nutrients and oxygen are cycled more effectively throughout the body. Sufficient blood circulation helps in accelerating the body's metabolism.

More importantly, enough oxygen reaching the body's vital organs optimizes and maximizes their functions. This beneficial result leads to a faster healing and recovery of the patient.

Fast Healing and Recovery

The combination of improved nerve function and blood circulation lead to the speeding up of a person's healing and recovery process. Through reflexology, metabolism is stabilized, cells are regenerated rapidly, and wounds heal faster. Furthermore, the pain relief effect of reflexology makes the recovery easier.

Eliminate Toxins

The improved flow of vital energy made possible by reflexology helps in the release and elimination of toxins in the body. When this happens, the body is prevented and protected from any disease and illness.

Reflexology is shown to improve the function of vital organs due to the reduction of toxins. Skin breakouts, such as acne and rashes, are experienced because of toxin release. Some people also experience diarrhea and increase in the frequency of fecal excretion. There have also been reports of improvements in the bladder function, especially for urinary tract issues.

Improvement in Emotional and Psychological Health

The practice of reflexology affects both the physical, emotional, and psychological health. Patients who have regular reflexology sessions are proven to have greater energy and stamina. Reflexology can enhance a person's overall mood. It is also known to reduce the effects of several psychological disorders such as severe depression and anxiety.

Aid in Women's Reproductive Health

Reflexology in pregnant women, taken with utmost precaution, is highly beneficial. Pregnant women, especially those in their last trimester, often experience edema. It is a condition in which the feet and ankles swell due to fluid retention. Foot reflexology helps in combating the symptoms of edema.

The therapy is also great for reducing the length of labor and the need for analgesics. There is also little to no chance of a post-partum depression. The recovery time of the woman's body after giving birth is also accelerated. Women suffering from PMS and menopause can benefit from regular reflexology sessions. The symptoms of PMS include excessive mood swings, irritability, fatigue, anxiety, and insomnia. During the occurrence of these symptoms, foot reflexology can help in alleviating them.

Consequently, the symptoms of menopause can also be eased through reflexology. Such symptoms are similar to those of the symptoms for PMS – in addition to hot flashes and chronic depression.

Prevent Foot and Ankle Injuries

Foot reflexology can strengthen the feet and the ankles. Stretching the muscles around these areas can prevent any future injuries and accelerate the recovery of such injuries. Constant sessions can help with joint pains and muscle soreness.

Flat feet is the condition in which ligament laxity in the feet causes the arch to collapse – thus causing a flat-shaped bottom part on the feet. Although this condition does not cause severe complications to the health, having flat feet is the reason for chronic foot and heel pain. Regular foot exercises, combined with foot reflexology, could focus on these conditions and eventually cure them.

Other Conditions that may benefit from Reflexology include:

- Allergies
- Arthritis
- Asthma
- Back Problems
- Blood Pressure
- Bowel Disorders
- Constipation
- Eczema
- Frozen Shoulder
- Hay Fever
- Insomnia
- Muscle Tension
- Neck Problems
- Sinusitis
- Thyroid Imbalance

Basic Reflexology Techniques

Proper basic reflexology techniques must always be implemented in order to achieve the benefits of reflexology optimally. The main reflexology techniques include: thumb walking and finger walking. The goal is to provide sufficient pressure into the reflex points using the thumb and fingers.
By using these techniques, anyone can learn the basic and proper way of practicing reflexology.

Thumb Walking Technique

The thumb walking technique is the easiest reflexology technique. It can be used for long periods of time without tiring the hands. This technique is great for foot reflexology. In this technique, the thumbs walk in a creeping motion through repetitive bending and unbending, using small movements in the area. Smaller movements of the thumb mean greater coverage on the reflex areas.

There is also a technique in choosing the part of the thumb to use for thumb walking. Put the hands together, at the palms, in front. Observe the tops of the thumbs. Touch both thumbs together at the top. At this point, the nails are slightly touching. The part of the thumb to use should be the part of the thumbs touching each other – located slightly on the inside of this part.

The execution of the thumb walking technique is quite simple. Place the thumb on the area to be massaged. Bend the thumb. Unbend the thumb, making sure that nothing else moves, while it stays in contact with the area. It would be noticed that the thumb has crept a little forward. With the unbent position of the thumb, a slight pressure can be applied on the area.

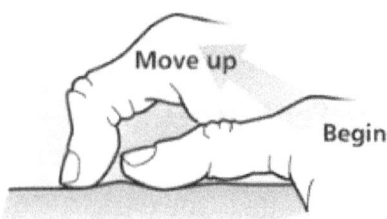

Thumb-walking: thumb bent at the first joint to take tiny steps with the outer edge of thumb making contact.
Source:
http://balancedwomensblog.com/tag/authorpaulinewills/

Finger Walking Technique

Finger walking technique has the same maneuver with thumb walking. Like the thumb walking technique, smaller movements can bring greater benefits. The fingers, more particularly the index fingers, are bent and straightened on the reflex area.

The finger walking technique is commonly used for hand and ear reflexology. It is because the reflexes in these areas are deeper than those on the feet. Usually, finger walking technique uses a circular motion to effectively apply firm pressure on certain reflex points. Slowly rotate the fingers into the reflex points for fifteen to thirty seconds in a clockwise manner. Then repeat for fifteen to thirty seconds in an anti-clockwise direction.

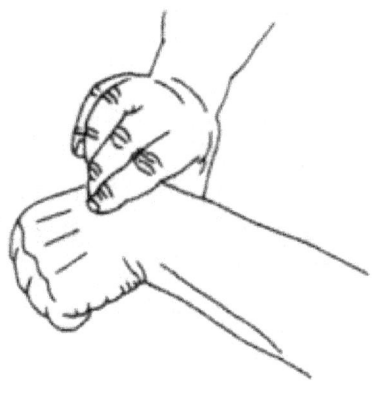

Other Techniques

Thumb walking technique and finger walking technique are the main reflexology techniques used by reflexologists. However, there are additional techniques used depending on the area of focus. These techniques include:

- Back and forth technique
- Ankle loosening technique
- Ankle stretch techniques
- Pin point technique

- Hook-in technique
- Basic holding technique
- Leverage techniques
- Toe twist and rotation
- Spinal twist
- Diaphragm tension relaxer

Conclusion

Reflexology is an Ancient form of therapy that promises total relaxation and peace. It is highly beneficial in restoring the body's inner balance. Most people know reflexology as an effective method of stress and tension release. This promising form of therapy also helps in reducing anxiety and depression.

Getting regular reflexology sessions is proven to provide a sense of well-being – for physical, emotional, and psychological health. Reflexology helps in giving a balanced state of mind, body, and spirit.

Indeed, the practice of reflexology can bring about a multitude of benefits and bodily effects. However, it is always important to keep in mind that reflexology should not be considered as a substitute form of treatment to any kind of illness. Reflexology only serves as another form of therapy combined with treatments and medications formally recommended by a medical personnel. Reflexology is not a standalone form of therapy to achieve wellness.

In addition to this, reflexologists cannot diagnose illnesses. Regardless of their ability to observe tension in the body, reflexologists are not authorized to name a certain health condition that a patient potentially has. In line with this, reflexologists are also prohibited to provide any kind of medication and treatment. The reflexologists' role in the healing process is to assist the patient in healing and recovery – not to provide the solution.

If a person is interested in undergoing reflexology, he must keep in mind that there are a few precautions and limitations to consider. Reflexology deals with sensitive reflex areas of the body. As such, it is best to consult a medical professional first before getting an appointment.

The effectiveness of reflexology varies from one person to another. A patient will not get the aforementioned benefits in just one session. Reflexology is a form of therapy that needs a little bit of time to get accustomed to. It would help for patients to communicate with their reflexologists and other patients if any concerns arise.